LYMPHEDEMA

Sentenced to
Life in Bed...

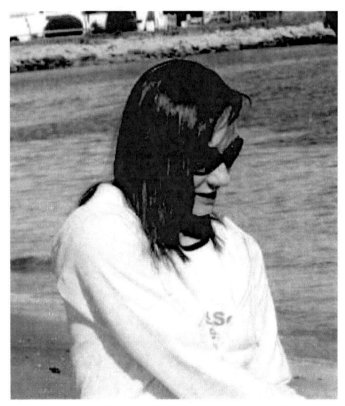

But I Escaped
By Karen M.Goeller, CSCS

LYMPHEDEMA
Sentenced to
Life in Bed…

But I Escaped

By Karen M. Goeller, CSCS

Dedicated to My Parents

To my dear Dad… You yelled at me to "get it checked" a hundred times over the course of a few weeks. You brought me to the hospital. You asked me if I needed anything when I was home recuperating. You were there for me. Then when I was, "back on my feet" it was your turn to be the patient and I was there for you, every day. I am not sure if you actually knew I was there sometimes. But I am willing to bet that you knew how much I cared for and appreciated you. You "saved the day" all my life, always solving problems, and rescuing me from the world. You saved my life. I only wish I could have saved yours.

And to my Mom… Who does everything for everyone, literally. You taught me when I was young that I "can do anything if I put my mind to it." Well, I used that advice over and over again, in my personal, school, and business life, beating the odds more than once. It was your work ethic, honesty, and strong mind that has inspired me all these years. Thanks Mom...

Contents

Sentenced to "Life in Bed"

No, really, I felt like I was being sentenced. I was told by every doctor that I would be bedridden for the rest of my life. Nearly twenty years later I can run up and down hills with my dog. Is it good for my leg? No, but I do it anyway because it's more fun than being bedridden! OK, I do come home and elevate my leg immediately after I take my dog out.

I have defied the odds more than once, but right now I will tell you about my lymphedema, life before cancer surgery, and my life after cancer surgery. I was an athlete, a coach, and a business owner. That life ended, or maybe it was just put on hold for a very long time. At least my life did not end as would have been the outcome without the cancer surgery.

The first year was hell, torture, and downright depressing. I went from being an athlete, gymnastics coach, fitness trainer, and business owner to being stuck in bed. My parents actually bought me my first TV with a remote control. I did not enjoy watching TV before my surgery, but then I was encouraged to watch TV when I was stuck in bed. What else was there to do? I could only read for so long. My friends and family worked so I did not have company throughout the day and I HAD to keep my leg elevated. I was bored and unhappy!

So I got up… And here's where I went from there…

A Bug Bite Gone Bad

It all started when I went to a local dermatologist. Actually, let me back up a bit. I had what looked like a bug bite on my leg, my right thigh to be exact.

I remember it being itchy, as most bug bites are, and then slowly turning into what looked like a typical brown mole.

A few months ago, I had a bug bite on my hand that turned into a small black mole. That one is a normal looking mole or freckle. So it does happen.

Little did I know that the mole on my leg was anything but typical. Over a few weeks the edges started to look dry and then part of the mole turned grey. The diameter of this mole started to grow and it became uneven, no longer round. Parts of it were raised. It became multicolored and ugly, but it was still pretty small in size. At the time, it was only a little larger than the eraser on a pencil in diameter.

All of this and I still did not take it seriously. Was I crazy or something? Looking back, I'd say that I was crazy not to get it checked. I did not have health insurance or much spare time on my hands.

I spent my days and evenings in the gym coaching gymnastics and then later at night I worked out in a local health club. I owned a gymnastics club at the time and worked long hours. I was tired sometimes, but I assumed it was from working so many hours and working out late at night. Owning a gymnastics club was a childhood dream come true. I did not want to do anything that would interrupt my work.

When I was 10 years old my gymnastics coach asked me if I had all of the money in the world what would I do with it. My teammates said they would buy big houses and cars. I responded, "I want my own gym." At 21 years old that dream was realized. I bought the gym where I worked for several years. There was no doubt I could handle the job. I did well growing the program. I opened in two different areas of Brooklyn, then grew enough to rent a large building to run my gymnastics program.

Most of my gymnastics success was after the cancer surgery. In other words, I did it while I was dealing with lymphedema.

Dad Warned Me

I was close to my Dad and usually listened to his advice. It was weird that I did not listen to him right away when it came to my health.

The weather was still warm enough where I had shorts on all the time. I assumed this little "mole" on my leg that turned ugly would go away, but my father knew better than that.

He noticed the mole on my leg and told me to get it checked. I actually ignored his advice. I cannot believe that I did not listen to him right away, but I didn't.

I did not have time or medical insurance. I just did not take it seriously. I guess I was young (age 24) and stupid. Another few weeks went by and every time my father saw me in shorts he told me to get the mole checked. Each time he reminded me to get to a doctor for this mole he became more and more serious. It got to a point when he yelled at me that I "better get it checked." He told my Mom to tell me to get it checked. She looked at my leg and called her friend for the name of her dermatologist. My Dad was really angry that I was not taking this small growth on my leg seriously.

Dad saved my life!

If it were not for my father yelling at me for a several weeks to find the time to get this mole checked I would not have gone and I would have died. I was close to my father and finally realized how serious he was when he yelled at me to get to a doctor. It's a good thing my Mom found a dermatologist. She took part in the life-saving bit too. Yes, I have had great parents who were on top of things.

I was a Work-a-Holic

I was young, seemingly healthy, and a true work-a-holic. Yes, I am a recovering work-a-holic. Throughout my childhood I watched my Mom dress up in nice clothes for work not to see her again until late at night or sometimes the next day. I knew she was doing something important and I knew she absolutely loved her work. That inspired me to find something that I enjoy doing and make it a career. My Dad worked more of a 9-5 job, so I saw him much more often than my Mom. He had tremendous pride in his work, but rarely worked late. So I have my parents to thank (or blame) for my work-a-holic tendencies!

I have always made it a point to take jobs where I loved the work, people, and environment. I easily left jobs where I was not happy. The majority of my jobs have been in the gymnastics industry, fitness industry, and I even spent two years working for the New York Police Department.

At the age of 21 my childhood dream of owning a gymnastics club was realized. As a young business owner and someone who absolutely loved her work, **how could I find time for a small mole on my leg?** I wanted to spend my time running my business, coaching gymnastics, and working out. Who knew this was a life-threatening situation? I certainly did not.

A Deadly Cancer

Malignant Melanoma can be deadly.
And I almost died from it. The doctors
said I was days away from death. They
were very surprised that it did not
already reach my lymphatic system
because it was large. The number they
told me to remember for future check-
ups was 1.85. I did not really know
what that number meant, but I did
remember it and every time I told a
doctor that number they seemed to be
surprised that it did not reach my lymph
nodes. Once a melanoma reaches the
lymph nodes it quickly spreads to every
organ and death is the result. I was
very lucky!

What Is Melanoma? According to the
website, **www.SkinCancer.org**,
Melanoma is the most serious form of
skin cancer. It is not the most common
of the skin cancers, but it causes the
most deaths. The American Cancer

Society estimates that at present, about 120,000 new cases of melanoma in the US are diagnosed in a year. In 2010, about 68,130 of these were invasive melanomas, with about 38,870 in males and 29, 260 in women.

Melanoma is a malignant tumor of melanocytes. Melanocytes are cells that produce the dark pigment, melanin, which is responsible for the color of skin. They predominantly occur in skin, but are also found in other parts of the body, including the bowel and the eye. Melanoma can occur in any part of the body that contains melanocytes.

Early signs of melanoma are changes to the shape or color of existing moles or in the case of nodular melanoma the appearance of a new lump anywhere on the skin (such lesions should be referred without delay to a dermatologist).

At later stages, the mole may itch, ulcerate or bleed. Signs of Melanoma include asymmetry, irregular borders, multi-colored surface, diameter greater than a pencil eraser, and it changes over time.

The most dangerous form of melanoma, nodular melanoma, also has the following signs. It is elevated, growing, and firm to the touch.

Metastatic melanoma may cause the following symptoms: loss of appetite, nausea, vomiting and fatigue.

Melanoma can metastasize and even spread to the brain. This is a serious medical illness.

The earliest stage of melanoma starts when the melanocytes begin to grow out of control. Melanocytes are found between the outer layer of the skin (epidermis) and the next layer (dermis). This early stage of the disease is called the radial growth phase, and the tumor is less than 1mm thick. Because the cancer cells have not yet reached the blood vessels lower down in the skin it is very unlikely that this early-stage cancer will spread to other parts of the body.

The behavior of the cells change dramatically when the tumor cells start to move into the epidermis and papillary dermis.

The next step is when individual cells start to acquire invasive potential. From this point on the melanoma is capable of spreading.

Next, the tumor reaches invasive potential, meaning it can grow into the surrounding tissue and can spread around the body through blood or lymph vessels. The tumor involves the deeper parts of the dermis.

There is an immunological reaction against the tumor which is judged by the presence and activity of the tumor infiltrating lymphocytes. These cells sometimes completely destroy the primary tumor which is the latest stage of the melanoma development. In some cases the primary tumor is completely destroyed and only the metastatic tumor is discovered.

Local Dermatologist Who Cared

I went to a wonderful dermatologist, Dr. Novick, in Brooklyn, NY. As I sat in the waiting room I saw a variety of people, young and old. I wondered why some of the people were there. Until I ended up there, I thought people only went to a dermatologist when they had acne problems. After sitting in the waiting room a while I figured I would look at some of the pamphlets they had for patient education. I picked up a skin cancer pamphlet and a melanoma pamphlet and looked at the photos. Before I was seen by the doctor I knew I had a melanoma on my leg. Even though I knew it was melanoma, I was not too concerned at that moment. I thought it would just be removed or treated with something like a cream. I assumed it would be taken care of in the office and that I would get on with my day, my life for that matter. I had no idea melanoma could be deadly. I was clueless!

So I went into the patient room and the doctor came in. I showed him my mole and his exact words were, "oh no, this has to come out." He had me lie back and he cut out the mole. He was good; I did not even feel him cut into my leg.

I thought it was over, dealing with this mole. Dr. Novick then told me it would be sent to the lab for a biopsy. The woman in the office said they would call me with the results in about a week. I left the office and thought it was all over. I really thought I could get on with my life and forget about the mole on my leg. Again, I had no idea melanoma could be deadly.

The Phone was Ringing

As I walked into my apartment immediately after the appointment with Dr. Novick the phone was ringing. It was the doctor's office. The woman on the other end of the phone said it is "serious." She said that I must be seen by an oncologist and they recommended a highly respected oncologist in New York City, Dr. Harris. This dermatologist's office called Dr. Harris at NYU Medical and made the appointment for me. The woman in Dr. Novick's office said she could get an appointment faster than I could. This was an urgent situation and it was important to have my records reviewed by Dr. Harris immediately.

The News

I was told by the woman in Dr Novick's office this may be "major cancer surgery." This was really NO JOKE. At that point, I knew it was very serious and learned that an ugly little mole could be deadly. I was scared and wanted to talk to my Dad.

I made the call to share the news. I think I even called him at work. I rarely called him at work. I remember telling my Dad and crying at the same time. I am not even sure when I told my Mom. I was overwhelmed with fear. I hardly cried at that time in my life and little scared me. I was a happy person and mentally tough.

Throughout my life my Dad was always the one who helped make a situation better. He saved the day every time, but he could not save me from the ordeal that I was about to face. My Dad could only hope that the doctors and surgeons would save my life.

My Dad was a strong man, there for everyone in their time of need. I never saw him cry or panic in a bad situation, but he did have feelings. He just wanted to be strong for all of us. He helped family members, friends, and neighbors with big and small problems. It's just who he was. When there was a problem, my father ran in to help, not out to survive.

Daddy's Girl

I was always close to my Dad. He was the one who brought me to gymnastics events, Broadway shows, out on his boat, and everywhere else he went. He always made sure my sister and I were safe, protected, and well cared for. We were a happy family of four that included family vacations, Sunday dinners, dining out, and celebrating holidays and birthdays together.

I found out six months later, at my Dad's funeral, that my Dad was crying at work when he told his friends that I was going to have major cancer surgery. I was a "Daddy's Girl." My Dad's friend, Ira, told me that my Dad said he wished it was HIM and not me dealing with cancer. And even as a young adult, my Dad was still the one I turned to for everything. It was pretty amazing; My Dad was not in perfect health, but he was there for everyone no matter how big or small the problem. Even when he was on dialysis and had to spend time on his own health care e was there to help.

I have talked about my Dad, but my Mom was just as concerned and wonderful as he was. She too has been the type of person to run and help whenever anyone needed her. She is still that way. Both of my parents have always been "givers."

My Friends

So there were **many days of crying and worrying**. I did not know what to expect. I called my best friend, Ilene, and she came over just a few minutes after I told her, just to keep me company. The following quote reminds me of my friend Ilene, "true friendship isn't about being there when it's convenient; it's about being there when it's not." To this day, I have no idea what she had planned for the day before she dropped everything and ran over to keep me company. We had some snacks as I told her all the details. I cried as I told her the news. Ilene almost cried and she reminded me she was there for me. I was her Maid of Honor at her wedding less than a year later.

I also told the parents of my athletes and my staff. I had several coaches that helped me run my gymnastics club. Everyone around me was truly warm and encouraging.

I knew that I had many people praying for me. And I believe their prayers helped. I was blessed to be surrounded by so many people that cared about me. Sometimes you do not realize how much people care for you until a life changing event is about to occur. I will always remember the people who helped me get through the days leading up to my surgery and the months and years after the surgery.

The Move

Going back to the first phone call with my Dad... When I told my Dad the news, he told me to move back home. I had a beautiful little apartment in Brooklyn, but we all knew I would not be able to live on my own after the surgery. Within two days I told my landlord the news and had several people helping to move me back to my parents' house on Staten Island. It was a beautiful house and I was back in my old bedroom. It felt good to be home, but I was not happy that I would be giving up my independence.

Our house had revolving doors for me and my sister over the years. My parents have always made sure we were OK and that included telling us to come home whenever we felt the need. Each of us moved back home at one time or another and our parents always made sure we were comfortable.

Sentenced to "LIFE IN BED."

My Mom came with me to meet with the oncologist, Dr. Harris in NYC. He was a highly respected doctor with tremendous experience and knowledge. His first words were, "**this is major cancer surgery**." He then went on to say, "This is no small surgery. It will change your life. You will be bedridden for the rest of your life. You will never work again. You will never have children." In other words, I was sentenced to "LIFE IN BED." I never cried so much in my entire life.

I had a lump in my throat that did not go away until after the surgery. My Mom's expression changed and I knew she became worried. And it was the first time I saw my Mom cry as much as she did. My Mom has always been mentally strong so when I saw her begin to cry I knew this was serious, life changing serious. The doctor repeated, "you will be bedridden for the rest of your life." My life really did flash before my eyes, but in slow motion. I thought of my gym and the faces of my athletes flashed through my mind. It almost seemed like a slide show of their faces. It was really strange. My mind went from my life to the doctor's words and back to my mental slide show repeatedly.

The doctor continued to talk telling us of the details of the surgery. Cut, biopsy, cut biopsy, etc. And then every other sentence seemed to be related to how my "life was over." It was the most horrible news I ever received. He said I would never work again several times. I just kept thinking of how much it would hurt to stop coaching, working out, and LIVING. I felt like I was losing a loved one. That loved one was me.

I was a very active young adult. After the horrible visit with this doctor we drove home, both still crying on and off. I really never saw my Mom that upset.

When I saw how upset both of my parents were in the days leading up to the surgery I knew that this was not a bad dream. It was reality. It was really happening. My life would NEVER be the same.

Who Knew It Could Spread?

And back to that horrible afternoon at the doctor's office... I know I already painted a picture of the meeting with Dr. Harris, but there is more. He told me and my Mom that the cancer may have already spread throughout my body. If that was the case I would not survive. It would be a quick goodbye. I am sure it hurt my Mom to hear that her young daughter may already have to say goodbye. For me, it was just unbelievable. I kept going back and forth with the life flashing before my eyes and the conversation with Dr. Harris. I was this strong young woman who could lift very heavy weights and I ate very healthy foods. How could my body be attacked by a cancer that would possibly kill me? I loved life at the time and did not want to hear that it could be over. I was in shock.

Dr. Harris explained that Melanoma can spread via the lymphatic system. If it gets into the lymph nodes it will spread to every major organ in my body. I was living a nightmare at age 24. The days before the surgery were very difficult for me, my parents, and my sister. Our family was scared. I think my friends and everyone at the gym was worried too.

In Less than a Week

So within less than a week I went from casually scheduling an appointment with a dermatologist to learning that I would need major cancer surgery and that I could die very soon. I was already very close with my parents, but this ordeal made us appreciate each other even more. I had a beautiful young nephew with whom I spent as much time as possible. I brought him to the baseball batting cages, babysat, and did everything I could to keep him happy. I was able to pick him up whenever I wanted and play any game with him. . I could no longer take him to the park, batting cages, or shopping. That suddenly ended. My young nephew probably did not know why I suddenly stopped playing with him, but he has always known how much I care for him. That nephew is now an adult. We worked together to complete the Swing Set Fitness books.

Surgery, Patient for Halloween

Each doctor I saw told me that I would be "**bedridden for the rest of my life**" and that I would "never work again." I just could not comprehend this. I believed the doctors, but thought how can this be? I just could not understand how someone as strong as I was could suddenly be bedridden. I heard the word bedridden more in one week than I did in my entire life. It seemed that every doctor I spoke with made it a point to use the word, bedridden.

I did all of the pre-op testing. I remember while I was waiting for one of the tests, a cat scan, other patients thought I was a nurse. I did not look like a patient and I certainly did not act like a patient.

My Dad was right there for me the day of the surgery. I remember my Mom being there, but not while I was being prepared for the surgery. My Dad sat with me and reminded me in his own way how much he cared for me. Before they gave me the shot to make me sleepy my Dad told me how scared he was before his open heart surgery and that I would come out of the surgery OK. He let me know how he and my Mom would be there for me every step of the way. And he tried to keep me as relaxed as possible by occasionally saying something a bit funny. He was not a joker, but my Dad did everything he could to keep me calm… and he did.

Bedside Manner

The surgeon was Dr. Lussier and there was a team of doctors that worked with him. Most of the doctors had absolutely HORRIBLE bedside manner. Dr. Hamm was the most compassionate of the bunch. Yes, they were trying to be honest, but was it really the right thing to do at that moment? I was crying as I was being wheeled in for surgery because I knew my life was either almost over or that I would be bedridden. The doctors kept reminding me that there was no way I would live a normal life ever again. Why did the surgeon have to tell me, as I was being put to sleep, that I would be bedridden for the rest of my life? Was that really necessary? Now what if I was the type to give up? Would the outcome have been different on that operating table?

Before I was asleep I remember the doctor bringing a radio into the operating room. I asked the nurse if that was normal. She said many surgeons do that. The doctor then started to draw on my leg where he would cut. He told me that there would be a skin graft where he was taking the melanoma from and that I would have another cut where the lymph nodes were coming from. And he reminded me AGAIN that I would be bedridden for the rest of my life. As they put the mask on me for the anesthesia, I was hysterical crying. I just did not want to be bedridden. And I certainly did not want to die!

Eight Hours Later

So about 8 hours later I remember being on the respirator. That was fun, sort of. Here's why. All I heard were the respirator machines and the nurses telling people to keep breathing. At first I really did not know if I was alive because I could not move and I did not know why I kept hearing nurses say, "keep breathing." It sounded a little like I was under water. I felt them tap my shoulder as they said, "keep breathing." It was really weird. I had to be reminded to breathe?

After a while I heard one nurse tell another that the respirators may not be recording the shallow breaths. And then the fun began. Yes, I was a wise-ass. A few times I intentionally breathed shallow just to hear them tell me to keep breathing. When I opened my eyes one nurse said, "you're awake already?" I could not respond with the tube down my throat. Having a tube down your throat is a miserable feeling. The next thing I remember is being wheeled to a room. I remember my throat being incredibly sore after they removed the respirator, but that went away pretty quickly.

Wheeled Out – It's NOT Over

So I was wheeled out of the recovery room and both of my parents were there. They stopped next to my Mom so she could say something to me. I remember my Mom being closer to the bed than my Dad. That was a switch, but either way, I was glad they were there! My Mom said a few times, "it's all over now." She meant the surgery part and that I could start healing now. I responded with, no it's not." She did not know why I was crying and responded that way. That obviously upset her because she thought I was telling her the cancer spread. I was really telling her I was going to be bedridden. I was thinking of the rest of my life and at that moment my Mom was thinking of the end of my life. I really scared her, but not deliberately. I thought I would have to lie in bed for rest of my life.

The doctors explained to my parents that they got all the cancer. When I was in the room my Mom told me they "got it all." She asked what I meant when I said it was not over. I reminded her that all of the doctors said I would be bedridden for the rest of my life. There's that horrible word again, bedridden. I was in the hospital for 8 days. My leg was wrapped and as wide as a tree trunk. I was not in a ton of physical pain, only emotional pain knowing my life was changed forever, over as I knew it. Or was it?

The Ride

So my Dad picked me up from the hospital and the ride home was sad and long. I was thinking of how my life had changed overnight. I thought I would never work again and that I would be bedridden or the rest of my life. I was scared and sad. I was also in shock that my life, as I knew it had ended. No more working out, no more coaching gymnastics, no more training fitness clients, no more playing with my young nephew, it was all over.

My Dad and I had to stop at a surgical supply store and order a compression stocking for my leg. The compression stocking had to be worn the rest of my life. After I was measured we got back in the car and the ride home was quiet. I am sure we were both exhausted from the horrible two weeks preceding that drive home, but we were both relieved that the cancer was gone. I do not remember much of the conversation we had as we drove, but I do remember the compassion in my Dad's eyes. I knew he felt my pain as he watched me get into the car, out of the car, and with each move I made.

Home Again

So I arrived home, eight days after major cancer surgery, a different person. I was no longer the big strong person that I was just 8 days before that. I was now weak and bedridden. When I arrived home I went straight to my bed. My leg was HUGE, probably the same measurement as my waist.

Oh no, there WAS some truth to what the doctors were telling me. I WAS bedridden. I was instructed to keep my leg elevated when not in motion. I had to stay off my feet unless it was absolutely necessary, such as to use the bathroom. And so, I did just that.

This was now the exact opposite of how I lived my life before the cancer surgery. I remember that I did not like to sit or watch television, or do anything of that sort. Now I was FORCED into a sedentary life, but at least I had my life, right?

That's not how I saw it. The day after I was home I took my first bath. (I was not able to stand in the shower or get the stitches and staples wet.) I had an exceptionally hard time getting into the tub, elevating my leg on the side of the tub, and doing everything else I tried to do.

Not being able to take a simple bath made me cry, it was depressing. I was a former athlete and I had trouble getting into the tub?!?! Seeing my staples, stitches, and the swelling was very upsetting even though I was the one who loved watching surgeries, I majored in physical therapy in college, I took countless health and science classes in college, and I was an EMT. I was intrigued by medicine and now I could not even look at my own leg.

I could no longer see the bulging quadriceps muscles and I felt like my leg weighed a ton. It hurt, mentally and physically.

I was Sad

I was more and more sad with each day, even though I was surrounded by people who loved me, I no longer had cancer, and the swelling was slowly going down each month. My leg looked like a tree trunk for months. I still had to remain in bed, could not work, and had no freedom. I still had a hard time bathing, could not stand long enough to make a sandwich, and was not in the gym. I was becoming depressed and did not tell anyone for a long time.

I finally told my friend Dean that I wished the surgery was too late. I told him that I wished I did not survive the surgery. He was sympathetic and told me it would get better each day. Dean was one of those friends who was there for me whenever I needed him. We worked together as coaches for many years and knew each other well. Dean was strong mentally and physically and he was compassionate. That was what I needed. He was the person who picked me up after an outpatient knee surgery the year before. Dean was right. It did get a little better each day. Even though I did feel a little better physically each day, I became depressed each time I realized I had limitations.

I remember one day, about 5 or 6 weeks after the surgery, I went to the post office and could not wait in line. I was not allowed to stand that long. I knocked on the door and told the postal worker that I recently had surgery and could not stand long enough to wait in line. He got me my stamps, but he said that was the only time I would be able to skip the line. I said to myself I will never be able to be independent again, another day of depression.

No one really knew how depressed I was. I was too embarrassed to tell anyone how difficult this was for me and how sad I felt. It did eventually get better, as I started to do more, but with each limitation there was sadness.

More Difficult Times

And then I went back to my gym. I was so happy to see my gymnasts and their parents again. The coaches were visiting me in the hospital and at home all along. When I arrived one parent found a chair for me to sit in so I could watch the workout. Being a spectator did not last for long. The parent then brought my chair to where my gymnasts were training.

I was not allowed to lift anything for one year. I started to coach gymnastics while sitting down. The joy only lasted a moment until a gymnast could not do what I asked her to do. She did not understand my instructions regarding skill on uneven bars. Before surgery I would have easily lifted her through the skill so she could feel what I was telling her, but the post-surgery I could not do that. I almost started to cry because I could no longer coach. I was so frustrated that I could not help my gymnast. She was making every effort to perform a skill on uneven bars and I just could not help her. The same thing happened with another gymnast. She also needed physical help with a skill.

A New Coach Evolved

Desperate to be able to coach again, I had to figure out better ways to explain skills. I had to learn more drills for the gymnastics skills my gymnasts wanted to perform. Dean always had great drills so that was a huge help, but I could not always take him away from the boys team. I spent the next several months learning every drill I could in order to help my gymnasts reach their goals. I traveled to other gymnastics facilities to see what their coaches were doing to teach their specific gymnastics skills.

As I became more involved in coaching, physically stronger, and more independent my depression was relieved. After using more drills for skills and conditioning exercises my gymnasts learned faster and started to win at competitions. I discovered that the best way to teach gymnastics was to assign drills and conditioning. My gymnasts really progressed so much faster, they had little to no overuse injuries, and they were strong.

This cancer surgery forced me to become a better gymnastics coach. It drove my career in a great direction. It is the reason I have such vast knowledge of gymnastics today. Even after I was able to stand (wearing a compression stocking) and lift (one year later) I continued to use drills and conditioning with my athletes.

My First Book

I became a better gymnastics coach. It was my turn to educate less experienced coaches. My first gymnastics book was all about gymnastics drills and conditioning. In my opinion, that was the best way to produce a strong and healthy gymnast.

I started writing after I was involved in an accident in 2001. It was not a gymnastics or car accident. A board fell on my head and I suffered permanent spinal damage. I wrote my first gymnastics book after the accident. That book was used by fitness and sports professionals to create countless fitness and gymnastics programs, including CrossFit.

For a second time in my life I was upset that I was not able to coach gymnastics. Writing a book was the best way for me to pass on my knowledge and stay involved.

I have continued to write books and articles ever since. I have published a series of gymnastics drills and conditioning books, swing set fitness books, several journals, and countless training programs. I have also written numerous articles on gymnastics, fitness, and health.

They Saved My Life

So yes, there were many people involved with saving my live... My Dad, the doctors. Mary Beth, a family member in the medical field, made sure the surgery was scheduled quickly and that everything was done right at the hospital. I have to say, many people really cared for me and I am fortunate to have so many wonderful people in my life.

The thing is, yes my life was "saved," but I was not actually living. After the surgery my day consisted of lying in bed and reading or watching TV, a very painful bath and then the compression stocking, eating a bit and then back to bed. Actually, I ate with my leg elevated in bed or in the living room for a long time. It was difficult to elevate my leg at the kitchen table in the beginning. Eventually, when I got my own apartment there were times I placed my leg right on the table as I was eating in order to elevate it.

Yes, alive, but what did I really do? I still owned a gymnastics club, but could not go to the gym for a long time. I did everything by phone and my staff members visited me often. I could not go out to eat because my BIG leg was in the way and too painful. I could not go to the moves because I could not stand in line and then there was no guarantee I could elevate it. I could not go shopping, not even Christmas shopping that first year, I could not go grocery shopping. I could not bring my nephew to the batting cages or play with him anymore. (That one hurt the most.) I could not go out with friends. The list could go on, but I'll spare you. I am sure you get the idea that there were numerous limitations on a daily basis.

So what COULD I do? I could hang onto the idea that I might one day be able to go to my gym.

I returned to my gymnastics club when the coaches called me several times each week to tell me that most of the team girls I coached were going to quit. The girls loved the other coaches, but they missed me. I went back to the gym about a month after the surgery. I sat in a chair just like the parents who watched their kids take classes. I was a spectator in my own gymnastics club and I did not like it. I was so upset because I could not really do anything in my own gymnastics club. I already told you how upset I was when I first attempted to coach again. That was extremely depressing and I almost broke down crying in front of the kids.

Once I was able to drive again I had some of my freedom. Things started to look up. I could not drive for very long because the stagnant position caused swelling. Remember, even in the compression stocking, the lymphatic fluid builds up. There is a constant battle between the swelling and the compression stocking.

There was still no LIFE or fun, but at least THERE WAS A GLIMMER OF HOPE. I would one day be able to do normal activities.

The Stocking

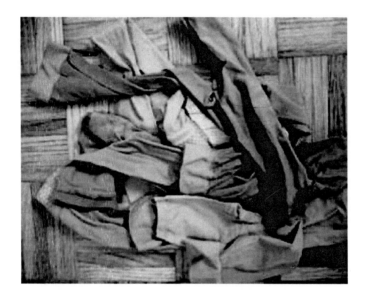

It hurts like hell when your leg starts to swell and the stocking squeezes your leg! I have felt nausea, dizziness, increased blood pressure, and other miserable symptoms when the fluid has built up. I sometimes still do.

Did you know that many compression stockings are made of rubber? Hmmm, makes you think of something else doesn't it? OK, all you men out there, STOP complaining! You should feel how miserable it is to have a huge piece of rubber over your entire leg! And the compression stocking stays on ALL DAY LONG.

Putting on a compression stocking is a job. It is not a quick or easy task. First, you MUST wear rubber gloves. The rubber gloves keep the oils from your fingers off the stocking. The oils from your fingers can ruin the compression stocking. The other reason for the rubber gloves is to grip and slide the stocking up your leg. First, you slip the compression stocking onto your foot and as much up your leg as it will go without actually pulling on it. Once you've done that you slide your hands up your leg so that the stocking slides up your leg. It is called donning. You continue to slide the stocking up a little at a time until it is at the top of your leg. It takes a long time to get good at putting on a compression stocking. I have even worked up a sweat in the past trying to put compression stockings on. For the open toe stockings there is a little slip that covers your toes so that the stocking glides over your toes easily.

These compression stockings are expensive, especially when you have to buy a few at a time. They range from $50.00 per pair to over $150.00 per pair.

I have been really happy that compression stockings have come a long way in the past twenty years. They now come in different colors, open or closed toe, thigh high, pantyhose, or with the waist attachment.

I have different ones for different activities and outfits. The ones I wear when I have a dress on are different from the ones I wear under my sweat pants for the gym. I even have a few with a lower than prescribed compression because there are days that I know I will not be doing much standing or walking.

When I first had the surgery there were very few compression stocking choices for me. I was prescribed full length, waist attachment, open toe, 40 mmHg. In recent years I discovered that I could use the thigh high with a silicone grip top, a more comfortable and less bulky stocking. The silicone grip beads do sometimes irritate my skin, but it's still better than the waist attachment. So glad I lost the bulky waist attachment! No more embarrassing bumps under my clothes. There was a thick strip of Velcro that extended from the stocking to go around the waist. I had to wear loose fitting clothes to hide the stocking so I rarely dressed in flattering clothing.

I am so glad the compression stocking companies now have more of a variety. Back in 1991 the only option for me was the big ugly tan one. It was so obvious that it was a medical stocking.

Even though there are many varieties of compression stockings now, I still will not wear shorts if I have a compression stocking on. So even during the summer, I wear sweatpants to the gym over my compression stocking. It's not comfortable, but neither is extreme swelling. People have asked the same question year after year" How can you wear sweat pants in this weather?" I tell them that I must wear the compression stocking. I do not want to ruin the stocking. I do not want to be seen with the stocking and shorts. It's just too ugly. So I avoid additional questions and other discomforts that go along with the ugly stocking. Fewer people ask questions when I wear sweatpants than would if they saw me in a compression stocking and shorts.

Fitness Article: Exercise with Lymphedema of the Leg

By Karen Goeller, CSCS

I am writing this article in response to a question from a fitness trainer on **how to exercise a client with lymphedema**. I am writing it from two points of view, as **a fitness trainer and as a patient** who has suffered with leg lymphedema since my 1991 cancer surgery. Before I discuss the effective exercises for lymphedema, I should explain what lymphedema is and what life is like with lymphedema.

I have been able to maintain my leg lymphedema pretty well because I understand the condition, I have listened to my doctors, I wear my compression stocking, I keep my leg elevated when not in motion, and I have extensive knowledge of exercise.

I have been disciplined with my daily care since the beginning. It is on my mind nearly every moment of every day.

Lymphedema is a very difficult thing to deal with and **must be maintained** all day long, every day. There is **no cure for lymphedema**.

I have had lymphedema in my leg since 1991. My lymphedema is the result of my lymph nodes being removed during cancer surgery. It is called secondary lymphedema.

I went from being a gymnastics coach, gym owner, and fitness trainer who exercised daily to being bedridden after my surgery. My life changed drastically.

I eventually went back to work, but with many physical limitations. I coached with my leg elevated and assigned more drills and conditioning exercises to my gymnasts because I could not lift them. (They ended up being better gymnasts as a result. In that way, it was a blessing in disguise.)

I learned how to maintain my lymphedema quickly. Several doctors told me that I would be bedridden for the rest of my life and that I would never work again after the surgery. They were partially correct because I was instructed not to get out of bed in the morning if my leg is still swollen from the previous day. It does not normally take days or weeks for the swelling to go down at this point, but there are still days that I remain in bed a few hours after waking up because of the swelling. I am able to eventually get up and go on with my day.

What is lymphedema? Here is the definition from VascularWeb.org... *"Lymphedema occurs when a clear fluid known as lymphatic fluid builds up in the soft tissues of your body, usually in an arm or leg. The lymphatic system consists of lymph vessels and lymph nodes that run through your body. Lymph vessels collect a fluid that is made up of protein, water, fats, and wastes from the cells of the body. Lymph vessels carry this fluid to your lymph nodes. Lymph nodes filter waste materials and foreign products, and then return the fluid to your blood. If your vessels or nodes become* *damaged or are missing, the lymph fluid cannot move freely through the system. The fluids can then build up and cause swelling, known as lymphedema, in the affected arms or legs. There are **two types of lymphedema**. Inherited lymphedema, sometimes called **primary** lymphedema, in which you are born lacking lymph vessels and nodes. The swelling usually appears during your adolescence and affects your foot or calf. A rare form of primary lymphedema develops in infancy and is called Milroy's disease. Acquired lymphedema, sometimes called **secondary** lymphedema, in which an injury to your lymphatic system causes lymphedema. It is much more common than primary lymphedema."*

What **types of exercise** can a lymphedema patient perform? That depends on the patient and whether they have medical clearance to exercise. Once medically cleared for exercise, the best exercise to reduce the leg swelling is swimming because the person is horizontal, the leg is in motion, and it is a non-impact exercise. The second best exercise for a person with leg lymphedema is riding a recumbent bike. It is also non-impact, it is a steady motion, and the legs are elevated slightly.

If the person with leg lymphedema is in good physical condition otherwise and they have the lymphedema under control they can use the elliptical machine. That is, if they can tolerate it from a fitness and medical standpoint. The elliptical is also non-impact because the foot remains on the pedals. It does not leave and strike a surface repeatedly. Make sure the lymphedema patient has permission from their doctor to exercise!

It is important to stay in motion and to perform **non-impact exercises**. An impact exercise is one where the foot leaves and strikes the surface repeatedly. A non-impact exercise is one where the foot remains on the surface such as the bike or elliptical.

Keep the person with lymphedema **OFF THE TREADMILL**. Walking and running cause the leg swelling to become MUCH worse because they are high impact. The swelling becomes dense / packed in from impact exercise.

Squats with light dumbbells are a better choice than walking lunges for someone with lymphedema. The walking lunge is an impact exercise and the squat is non-impact. **It's all about keeping the body in motion without any impact.**

The more severe the swelling, the more difficult it is to deal with. In my experience, it can take over an hour with the leg elevated before the swelling even BEGINS to go down and several days or weeks of elevation for it to drain more completely. **The longer it is swollen, the longer it will take to drain**.

Unless their doctor has instructed otherwise, people with leg lymphedema should be wearing a compression stocking and sleeping with the leg elevated every night. A compression level should be prescribed by the doctor. The stockings come in various compression levels, open or closed toe, and hip attachment or rubber beads to keep it up. I have used the Sigvaris stockings because they are made really well. Back in 1991 there were very few choices. The compression stockings were very thick (rubber) and an ugly tan color. Now there are some compression stockings that actually look like pantyhose. That is an amazing breakthrough for those of us who want to look "normal" when wearing a dress or skirt. They even come in other colors now! I was truly thrilled to see the more sheer styles of compression stockings.

Keep in mind that the patient MUST be cleared to begin exercise. If they begin to exercise before the doctor allows them to exercise they can cause permanent damage to the lymphatic system. **My doctors told me to wait one full year after my surgery before I was allowed to exercise.** I waited 10 months and just couldn't stand it any longer. Not being allowed to exercise was extremely difficult for me because I spent a lifetime in the gym. Again, make sure the lymphedema patient has FULL medical clearance to exercise.

When a person with lymphedema is not in motion and does not have a compression stocking on their leg, they **MUST keep their leg elevated** in order to prevent swelling. Something as simple as waiting in line at the grocery store can cause enough swelling to keep a person in bed the next day. I am serious.

The swelling can begin in less than a minute when standing still or sitting without the leg elevated. It is truly a challenge every minute of every day to keep the leg from swelling. Those close to lymphedema patients must be patient and considerate. If lymphedema is not controlled it can end up being **elephantitis**. Yes, that is a real medical condition and it is **very** serious.

There are lymphedema support groups throughout the USA. The National Lymphedema Network has plenty of useful information, www.lymphnet.org.

By Karen Goeller, CSCS

Twenty Years Later

So here I am, twenty years later, sitting with my leg elevated as I write this. I am still cancer free. As a matter of fact, five years ago the doctors congratulated me. The first time a doctor said, "Congratulations!" I wondered what he meant so I asked him. I knew it was not my wedding anniversary or any other personal anniversary that week or month.

The doctor said, "It's been over 15 years since your cancer surgery. You are cured." I remember being so happy and a very relieved. It was as if a weight had been lifted off my shoulders. I had to go call my Mom and a few friends to share the news. The doctor explained that in the medical world fifteen years out is considered CURED, the cancer is not expected to return. Now that's HUGE!

You'll appreciate just how amazing this is when you read this... Just before my cancer surgery the medical research on malignant melanoma stated that a patient had **a 95% chance of dying within the first five years**. I'll admit, I was scared for the first few years, but I also knew how to improve and maintain my health. And at the five year mark, I knew I already beat the odds. I think the fact that I ate healthy foods and exercised appropriately (as soon as I was allowed by the doctors) were the reasons I continued to improve and maintain my health.

I know that your diet directly affects your health and have known that since I was a child. In grammar school (6th grade) health class we learned the basics about nutrition and medical conditions. That class was the reason I became so interested in health and nutrition.

So again, here I am twenty years later. You may think, why the complications with lymphedema all these years later if the cancer was removed and I am considered "cured?" Although the cancer was removed and I am now cured of the cancer, **my lymph nodes were also removed** during the surgery. The fact that my lymph nodes were removed is the reason I suffer from secondary lymphedema.

Secondary Lymphedema cannot be cured. It can be maintained, but not cured. Lymphedema is a life-long battle that I must fight. I've been told that it will get worse with age. Yes, it is annoying, painful, and it just plain sucks at times, but I do have my life. And I am pleased with that. My life is full now and I am able to live INDEPENDENTLY, something I thought would never be possible. Remember, I was told a few days before the surgery that I would never work again, would never have a family, and would never live a normal life. The doctors were wrong!

On a Daily Basis

Most people wake up and they can just jump out of bed. Not me. I have not been able to do that on a daily basis ever since October 31, 1991, the day of my cancer surgery. Yes, my surgery was on Halloween day. Before I tell you about my day, or at least the part that is affected by lymphedema, I will tell you about my nights. By the end of the day, when I am headed to bed my leg is often swollen. If it's not swollen, it hurts like hell from being in a compression stocking all day long.

I prepare a meal that is fast so that I can get off my feet quickly. It is often eggs, salad, pasta, quinoa, or fish and my meal always includes plenty of vegetables. After I eat dinner, I use rubber gloves to remove the compression stocking. I elevate my leg as I unwind for the night. When I go to bed, I must sleep with my leg elevated on two pillows so that the swelling will drain by the time I wake up in the morning. My leg is not always drained by the morning so I must remain in bed until the swelling goes down.

When I Wake Up

I sometimes toss and turn throughout the night so my leg does not remain on the pillows all night. The first thing I do when I wake up in the morning is look at my leg to check for swelling. I've had to do that since the surgery. If my leg is still swollen or painful from the day before I cannot get out of bed.

Well, I CAN get up if I want to, but the swelling would build day by day. Think of a snow storm. Now think of another snow storm the next day. The snow did not melt from the first storm. Now you have twice as much snow. It will take much longer for two days worth of snow to melt than if you only had one snow storm.

It is the same idea with fluid buildup in a leg with lymphedema. If you do not allow the leg to drain from one day of swelling and you continue to allow the swelling without letting it drain you end up with a severe backup of lymphatic fluid. And when you have a few days of lymphatic fluid in your leg it feels like it is really packed in. It is very painful and can be very dangerous. It feels like I have several ankle weights strapped onto my leg. Lymphatic fluid is not the same as swelling form water. Diuretics are not the answer for lymphedema.

Eventually a person with lymphedema could end up with a permanent condition known as elephantitis. I choose to remain in bed until the swelling goes down each day to prevent serious complications.

I am sometimes in bed another two hours waiting for the swelling to go down. When I stay in bed in the morning like that I make sure my leg stays on the pillows. That is the only way to reduce the swelling on a daily basis.

Yes, there are therapies and machines that reduce the swelling, but I usually maintain my lymphedema well enough that I do not need to use the expensive medical supplies.

Now you must be thinking, "I could never stay in bed another two hours." Well, I bet you would if was your only choice! And when you consider the fact that I was originally sentenced to "Life in Bed" this is not a bad alternative. Yes, I am bed-ridden some mornings, but it's not as bad as the doctors described because I am able to live a full life once I am up for the day.

I Am Unreliable, No Really, I Am

The lymphedema is the reason I am
unreliable in the mornings and early
afternoons. I never schedule anything
in the early part of the day in case I am
stuck in bed waiting for my leg to drain.
Yes, that puts a damper on life. And
yes, I do miss out on so much, but
remember it's nothing compared to the
alternative. I almost lost my life.

Yes, I was sentenced to "Life in Bed."
And I have been paying ever since. But
when you compare the way the doctors
predicted how my life (or lack of life)
would be, I have lived a dream life. I
was not expected to ever enjoy life
again. But guess what, I am enjoying
life more now than I have in years!

I have accomplished so much since the
cancer surgery and I am able to live an
almost normal life. When you compare
how I lived before the surgery to how I
have lived after the surgery, my life

became very difficult. Is the glass half empty or half full? It's not that difficult an answer in this case... is it? I like my life right now.

I was an athlete, coach, and business owner before my surgery and had absolutely no limitations. I was super strong mentally and physically. I even tried out for the American Gladiators show a month before my surgery. I ran 1/10 of one second too slow twice so I was eliminated. My Dad even saw me running on the news that evening when they covered the Gladiator tryouts. He could not believe it was me they showed running. I thought they were going to show my friend Megan because they interviewed her.

I did not decide to go to the Gladiator tryouts until midnight the night before. I did well considering the fact that I did not train or plan for it and I had cancer in my body. I was planning on doing speed drills so that I could improve my running speed, but I was sidetracked by cancer surgery. The pull-ups and push-ups were extremely easy for me. I went from being able to squat 225 pounds and doing pull-ups with weights tied around my waist to being a cancer patient overnight.

Best Friend, Worst Enemy

Let me tell you how my typical day goes. Once I finally do get out of bed, I am forced to make a quick breakfast. I cannot spend an hour making steel cut oats each morning, which is really my preferred breakfast. I use faster-cooking steel cut, 5 grain, or organic oatmeal. No, I do not use the instant stuff in a package. The instant stuff is often loaded with sugar.

Remember, if I stand too long without a compression stocking on my leg it will begin to swell. It only takes a few minutes for the swelling to begin. Lymphedema could ruin my day before it even starts. The dilemma, I do not put the compression stocking on until after my shower, but I like to eat when I wake up. I am really supposed to put the stocking on before I get out of bed in the morning, but I prefer to take showers in the morning so I do not put the compression stocking on until after my shower.

As you can see, the lymphedema is on my mind from the moment I wake up, through breakfast, and then ALL day long.

Lymphedema has become my best friend and worst enemy. I think of it all day long, make sure it does not get out of hand, and I take care of it when there are complications.

It Never Leaves Me

OK, I admit, I do not wear the full length 40mmHg compression stocking EVERY day. I sometimes feel like I can get away with the 30mmHg knee high compression stocking. (I really can't, but I like to think I can.) It is not the best idea, but sometimes the full length stocking is so hot and painful, especially during the summer.

On days I wear the knee high compressions stocking, the fluid does not build in my lower leg, but it does remain in my knee and thigh. The fluid causes knee pain and it is really unsafe to allow any fluid to build up at all. It is really not a good idea to go with the smaller stocking, but again, it is just so hot during the summer. I usually go with the smaller stocking if I know I will not be doing that much standing.

All right, busted! There are days when I just do not wear ANY compression stocking. After the surgery I thought I would never see the day. Now I'm a rebel. I'll only do that if I know I can elevate my leg and I will not be forced to stand. If I know I'll be home most of the day I allow my leg to breathe. Yes, I do sometimes pay for it when I go without the stocking and my leg swells. It is painful when my leg swells, it could be dangerous, and it is pretty damn ugly. So why do I do that? I go without the compression stocking because I want to feel "normal" as often as possible.

A Bit Stressful

Did you ever get stuck in traffic or stuck waiting in line at the grocery store and you suddenly realize that you must be somewhere else or that you must use the restroom? It's the same type of stress or urgency that I feel when I am forced to stand in line at the store and I feel the lymphatic fluid building. It's stressful knowing my leg is swelling when I cannot do anything to change my situation. You know you need the stuff in your shopping cart, but you also know that you will regret getting in that line. I run errands at night so that my leg will have time to drain while I sleep.

If I do too much standing during the day it is not only painful, but the swelling could get really bad before I have a chance to elevate my leg. When my leg swells during the day I know it will be hours before I get a good chance to drain my leg. That is stressful because the longer it is swollen, the longer it takes to drain.

I can actually feel the fluid building up inside my leg when I stand for more than a few minutes.

I know the only thing I can do to minimize the swelling is to get off my feet and elevate my leg. It's not always convenient to do that. Now imagine having those thoughts all day long, the stress of knowing that you must get out of the situation or you will regret it for a day or even a few weeks, depending upon how bad the fluid buildup is.

No One Knows

Dealing with the swelling is truly stressful. And to make matters worse, no one I know has a clue what it is like to feel this sense of urgency ALL day long. Lymphedema is literally on my mind every day, all day, and that will never change.

I am fortunate to have some friends that understand how important it is to elevate my leg. My wonderful friends Dale and Michael immediately found a way to make me comfortable in their home. They had me elevate my leg as soon as I walked into their house. They were very accommodating and understanding. Unfortunately Dale and Michael moved out of state so I do not see them anymore. It is always a relief when the people around you make every effort to help you take care of your health and make you comfortable.

Of course my family knows why I elevate my leg. It doesn't faze them anymore when I put my leg on the arm of the couch or pull over an extra chair for my leg. It's how I have lived for twenty years.

It's strangers that get annoyed with me. Once I was visiting my Dad in the hospital and had my leg on a chair. He was in intensive care and only one person was allowed to visit him at a time. When I left the waiting room to see my Dad in intensive care someone made a remark about my leg being up on a chair. I looked very young and healthy so they just did not understand. When I returned my Mom told me what happened and she told the ignorant person that I HAD to elevate my leg as a result of a surgery. It was nice to know that she stood up for m. It was a little upsetting to me because of the limitations I had and how I had to live my life. It was now my Mom's turn to go in to see my Dad in intensive care.

My family was worried about my Dad and we had strangers at the hospital commenting on how I had to sit in the waiting room. As if the stress of my Dad being sick wasn't enough. Some people will NEVER get it that there are people in this world that MUST deal with medical issues.

Another time I was in the movies and had to place my leg on the space between the seats in front of me. The movie employee asked me to move my leg and I had to explain to him that my leg swells from a surgery. That has happened more than once. I always make sure no one is sitting right in front of me so that my foot does not hit anyone's head. The swelling and dealing with lymphedema is not as bad as it was in the beginning.

You see, I look very healthy. When a stranger sees me elevating my leg, they assume I am being disrespectful or lazy. If they only knew!

I was told that the lymphedema would get much worse when I get older. Now there's something to look forward to!

I Look Healthy

Why do I look so healthy? Because I eat good food and I exercise often. I never eat from fast food places, (I just cannot call them restaurants.) I eat plenty of fruits and vegetables, and I try to stay away from processed foods. That's not very easy, but I do make an effort.

I eat most of my meals at home. I know exactly what is in my food, I know it is prepared properly, and I can elevate my leg when I eat.

I eat fruit 4-5 times a day, each time a different fruit. I think that helps tremendously. I eat a few servings of vegetables each day too. And I eat plenty of whole grains and nuts. People often ask if I am a vegetarian. I am not, but I hardly eat meat. I do eat fish and eggs often.

I also drink plenty of fluids, usually water, tea, and almond milk. Alright, I do occasionally drink a decaffeinated coffee after dinner, maybe once every few months.

Staying hydrated helps tremendously with your health, so make sure you are drinking plenty of water! Did you know (unless directed otherwise by your doctor) that you should drink a minimum of half your bodyweight in ounces each day? For example, if you weigh 100 pounds you should drink a minimum of 50 ounces a day. You must drink more on days you sweat profusely.

Mild dehydration causes fatigue, loss of concentration, dizziness, and a host of other problems. A person can literally die of dehydration. Stay hydrated! I have written an article on dehydration and it is posted on my website, **www.KarenGoeller.com**.

Even with the Stocking

Even when I do wear the compression stocking, my leg attempts to swell. The compression stocking just prevents it from getting huge. There is a constant battle going on between my leg lymphedema and the compression stocking. And that battle hurts.

It is very painful when the fluid is building up in my leg and pressing against my skin and then the compression stocking squeezes my leg. It's a burning sensation and a heavy feeling, as if I have cement shoes and socks. It becomes difficult to lift my leg to take a step. Now imagine this pain and discomfort nearly all day long. Imagine a rubber band on your wrist that is too tight. Now imagine you have them along your entire arm or leg and you cannot take them off all day long, maybe as long as 10-14 hours. That's what a compression stocking feels like, not pleasant.

Just because the compression stocking minimizes the swelling in my leg does not mean there is no extra lymphatic fluid build-up in my body. One doctor recently told me that the fluid could build up in my torso and my other leg before my body rids it. It makes sense. My leg attempts to swell so the fluid must go somewhere. Even though all of the lymphatic fluid is not staying in my leg, the fluid may cause problems elsewhere in my body. I get nauseous and for the first year I ran a fever when the lymphedema got bad. I have been told that I have a good poker face. I almost never complain about my aches and pains and I push myself to get through my day. It's OK. I choose to be productive, social, and happy.

Leg lymphedema can cause serious medical problems that I want to avoid.

From the website, **www.lymphnet.org**, *"When lymphedema remains untreated, protein-rich fluid continues to accumulate, leading to an increase* of swelling and a hardening or fibrosis of the tissue. In this state, the swollen limb(s) becomes a perfect culture medium for bacteria and subsequent recurrent lymphangitis (infections). Moreover, untreated lymphedema can lead into a decrease or loss of functioning of the limb(s), skin breakdown, chronic infections and, sometimes, irreversible complications. In the most severe cases, untreated lymphedema can develop into a rare form of lymphatic cancer called Lymphangiosarcoma (most often in secondary lymphedema)."

Daily Care Beyond the Stocking

Besides wearing the compression stocking there are many things that must be considered daily. In addition to dealing with the lymphedema, I must take precautions as I go through my day.

The one thing that most people do not understand is that I must be careful with germs. It not recommended that I shave the leg or cut the cuticles on that foot. I do not usually shave my legs, I wax. It's OK; they look better after waxing than shaving anyway. At least with wax there are no sharp razors or cuts to worry about. But if you go to a professional for waxing, be careful with the temperature of the wax. I was burned by wax twice and that could be dangerous.

I have to avoid athlete's foot and clean between my toes carefully. I must make sure I do not step on anything that would cut my foot or cause infection. That is why I always wear something on my feet. I even wear slippers or flip-flops in my house. I never walk around barefoot.

The research I read right after my cancer surgery, and the information the doctors confirmed, was that germs could cause serious complications with lymphedema. An infection could send me to the hospital. Great, a place where I can pick up MORE germs!

After my surgery it was recommend that I carry antibiotics, alcohol swabs, and a first aid kit to take care of any cut or other mishap immediately. I did do that for the first year. Keeping a first aid kit with me was annoying. I do still carry antibacterial wipes and a few Band-Aids, just in case. OK, I admit it, there is a first aid kit in my car.

You would not believe how much there is to think about when doctors tell you to avoid germs! It's insane! Can you spell GERM-APHOBE? I wash my hands often, use Lysol in my house to kill viruses on surfaces, and always make sure my food is prepared properly.

Since my lymph nodes were removed, I have fewer "filters" than anyone whose lymph nodes were not removed. In other words, dealing with bacteria, virus, or other issues could be problematic. It's a real pain in the neck to worry about germs and swelling all of the time, but again, the doctors saved my life with the surgery.

The Texas Hospital

Here's a horror story... I ended up in the hospital while I was working in Texas. That was NOT fun! I started to get shooting pains going up my leg. A co-worker drove me to the hospital.

I was at the hospital for a few days with what they thought could be a blood clot, an infection, or some other lymphedema complication. The doctors really did not know how to deal with a lymphedema patient with sharp pains in the leg. You know what they did? They tied me to a board, literally. Then they took a large needle and stuck it into the vein on top of my foot, and then they tilted the board so I was nearly upside down. How barbaric was that?!?!

The doctor said he had to inject dye to see if there was a clot in my leg. Do you know how painful it was to have that huge needle stuck into my foot? That hurt!

I was in Texas because I was coaching at the Karolyi Gymnastics Camp. I worked for Olympic Coach Bela Karolyi for seven summers until it became too difficult for me health-wise. Bela and Martha Karolyi were the coaches of Nadia, Kim Zmeskal, and many other Olympic gymnasts. I truly loved coaching at their ranch. I learned so much, made many friends, and was able to do what I love doing most... coach gymnastics. Working for Bela Karolyi was the highlight of my gymnastics career! He was very friendly and generous with his knowledge. He allowed me to watch him train his Olympic gymnasts each summer.

I just could not deal with the standing all day, even though I was wearing my compression stocking. And did I mention that it was over 100 degrees on most days?!?! It was awfully hot with that compression stocking on, and then I had sweatpants on top of the stocking. NOT comfortable, but I loved every minute that I was coaching at the ranch. It was truly a happy and productive place.

Not Going Away

Constant elevation, compression stockings, germs, late mornings... These are things the average person does not think about every day.

When you look at each individual issue with lymphedema it does not seem all that bad. When you combine all of these factors together, and the fact that the lymphedema patient must think of these things all day long, you realize it is a major responsibility. And it is not going away any time soon.

Lymphedema is not cured. The lymph nodes that were removed will never grow back or be replaced. My lymphatic system was compromised permanently, but I do have my life.

I have a small window of opportunity every day to be productive and enjoy life. During that time I take my dog to the beach, ballroom dance, coach clients, write articles, promote my books, and spend time with friends and family. Yes, I have fewer hours to LIVE, but I am doing more LIVING now than I have in years.

IT'S ALL GOOD… I love my life now… I have a wonderful family and great friends. I enjoy my free time and I enjoy my consulting work.

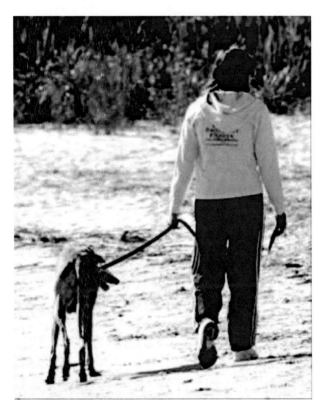

Hope it Helped

If you have lymphedema, I sincerely hope this book helped you prepare for or deal with your medical issue. Always remember to try to get out there and live a full life. Do not hesitate to contact me if you feel I can help you deal with lymphedema.

About the Author

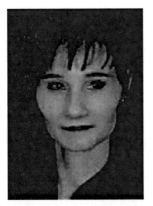 Karen Goeller has educated thousands in the fitness and gymnastics industries with her books, articles, and in person. She has been training athletes since 1978 and adults since 1985. Karen Goeller is the author of more gymnastics books than anyone in the USA.

Karen started writing books after she was involved in an accident in 2000 and suffered permanent spinal damage. She stopped coaching gymnastics and left her advertising job. To remain involved in gymnastics and fitness, Karen turned to writing. "I felt like I had a ton of information in my head that was not being used. I knew it was the perfect time to pass on this knowledge and writing books was the perfect avenue."

Karen Goeller's first book, "Over 75 Drills and Conditioning Exercises" was used to create countless successful fitness and gymnastics training programs. Her books have been called the "most useful on the market."

Karen's most recent books are the Swing Set Fitness books. They were completed with Brian Dowd, Karen's nephew, who is a physical education teacher. It wasn't until the Swing Set Fitness books that Karen started to make good progress with her physical rehabilitation. Karen shared, "I finally feel like myself again. I knew I was getting stronger, mentally and physically." When asked if she is healed from the accident, Karen replied, "I am still injured, but that no longer defines me."

Karen has produced NY State Champions, National TOPS Team

Athletes, and Empire State Games Athletes. Three National Champions are from Karen's gymnastics club. This success was after her 1991 cancer surgery. The cancer surgery was a success, but Karen was left with **lymphedema** in her leg. She was forced to keep her leg elevated or in motion 24/7 and in a compression stocking.

Karen Goeller and her athletes have been featured in the media since the 1990's. He has appeared on Good Morning America, GoodDay NY, Eyewitness News, and NY Views (old show) among others. They have also been featured in The NY Times, NY Newsday, Brooklyn Bridge Magazine, and Interview Magazine, and most of the Brooklyn, NY neighborhood newspapers. More recently Karen has been featured on Erin Ley Radio, Lynn Johnson Radio, I Run MY Body Radio, Late Night with Johnny Potenza TV, Talkin' Health with Joe Kasper Radio, the Coast Star, Asbury Park Press, Observer/Reporter, Staten Island Advance, and Inside Gymnastics Magazine. Karen has worked for world famous Olympic coach, Bela Karolyi and was his first female camp director.

Before earning her BA Degree, Karen's education included training as an EMT, Physical Therapist, and Nutritionist. She has had certifications such as EMT-D, Nutritional Analysis, Fitness Trainer, many USAG certifications, and the NSCA-CSCS certification.

References

1. SkinCancer.org
2. Mayoclinic.com
3. wikipedia.org
4. emedicine.com
5. cancernews.com
6. lymphnet.org
7. foryourlegs.com

Books by Karen Goeller

- Fitness on a Swing Set
- Fitness on a Swing Set with Training Programs
- Swing Set Workouts
- Gymnastics Drills and Conditioning Exercises
- Handstand Drills and Conditioning Exercises
- Gymnastics Drills: Walkover, Limber, Back Handspring
- Gymnastics Conditioning for the Legs and Ankles
- Gymnastics Journal: My Scores, My Goals, My Dreams
- Most Frequently Asked Questions about Gymnastics
- Fitness Journal: Goals, Training, and Success
- Strength Training Journal
- Gymnastics Conditioning: Five Conditioning Workouts
- Gymnastics Conditioning: Tumbling Conditioning

www.KarenGoeller.com

CPSIA information can be obtained at www.ICGtesting.com
Printed in the USA
LVOW111857120612

285799LV00001B/388/P